Everyday I

In

Emotional Intelligence

A Caribbean Perspective

Terrin Jaiga Callender

Amala Luncheon, Ph.D.

Table of Contents

Dedication

To the person who is self-aware enough to own the role
they play, even if it is not the role they wanted.

Acknowledgment

Sometimes you find yourself in the midst of a storm. You do not control the elements but if you align yourself as you should, you will be left standing after the storm has passed. The idea for this book had its genesis in one of those "What to do with your dissertation?" searches.

I am grateful to Dr. Jeannine Bennett of Vision to Purpose for putting this on my list of things to do, her nudge was the tipping point. Like everything in life, there should be a balance to maintain equilibrium, the world is still at odds over whether the screeching halt caused by the Covid-19 pandemic was good or bad. It really depends on the lenses you are viewing it from. If climate change and emissions are high on your agenda, then you see the good. I think we all empathize and see the bad in the lives lost.

However, the opportunity presented a chance to reset because we had literally stopped moving, and needed to figure out the next steps. Some of us got onto a different but adjacent path. We acquiesced to the energy transmuted by the imposed change and seized the opportunity to collaborate on a project we find both interesting and relevant in the now.

We are incredibly grateful to GBM Productions for the hospitality and facilitation of the recording.

About The Authors

Terrin Callender is best known as Jaiga in Trinidad and Tobago and the Caribbean. An artist, radio personality, songwriter, father of two, and all-around creative genius, the soca lover and undying patriot has given most of his life to the culture of Trinidad and Tobago. In a concerted effort to entertain, educate, and inform, he takes the time to understand subjects and relay them to his audience in a format they appreciate. Recognized for his "Great is the Artform" brand, Terrin is willing to lend his support to anyone who can benefit from his advice and expertise.

Dr. Amala Luncheon is a management professional who consistently strives to marry her love of Caribbean culture with academia. Having worked across different industries in three countries, she has developed an appreciation for the soft skills that make organizations and social interactions seamless. Dr. Luncheon, who holds a Ph.D. in Management with a specialization in Leadership and Organizational Change, is a systems thinker and creative problem solver who applies a holistic approach to problem-solving, which is a highly valued skill in today's volatile, uncertain, complex, and ambiguous environment.

Foreword

Born and raised in Guyana, Amala Luncheon honed her career skills in Saint Lucia including coordinating the Caribbean Soca Monarch for a decade. She has spent the past eleven years of her life in the USA and completed her Ph.D. in Management, with specialization in Leadership and Organizational Change.

Recognizing a gap in knowledge about "emotional intelligence," from her dissertation work, Luncheon now resident in New Jersey, has written a book on the subject from a Caribbean perspective.

Co-authored with popular Trinidad & Tobago radio personality and soca artiste Terrin "Jaiga" Callender, this publication addresses the ability to understand one's emotions, how to control those emotions, understand the emotions of others and how to make emotions work for you, whether when relating to family, with co-workers, fellow parishioners in church or any other form of social interaction.

The concept of "emotional intelligence" was developed in the 1990s. "Everyday lessons in Emotional Intelligence - A Caribbean Perspective" will help you reminisce while you learn.

Peter Ray Blood

Former T&T Guardian Features Editor

Introduction

Jordan, Jackson, or Pippen?

Emotional intelligence is an essential trait for the general populace to possess to be effective during interactions with each other and successful in society at large. Soft skills are becoming as crucial as making quotas are in retail stores. The fact that there is a paucity of research on this topic in the Caribbean could allow for a contribution to positive social change for organizations. I discovered both the lack of research on the topic and an accompanying low understanding of it at the managerial level when I was conducting doctoral research and wanted to situate the topic in the Caribbean. The implications for positive social change include the potential benefit to human resource managers, leaders, managers, and employees of organizations as the findings may provide insight into how learning emotional intelligence can positively impact human interaction in general.

When Terrin and I sat in a creative session to begin work on this project, we started talking about everyday stories and interpersonal relationships. Of course, that is where you see most of the opportunities for growth as it relates to emotions. Think about your colleagues at work. Think about the lines at the bank. Think about your interactions with the medical professionals. I like to say that people pretend well.

1

However, they can only do it for so long. At some point, if you do not have a grasp on self-awareness, your lack of emotional intelligence will glare like a spotlight. Terrin said something that at the moment, my Pentecostal heart quivered, and I thought – 'a word'!

The 'word' that was a revelation to me was that in life, we all want to be the best at what we do. Not only do we want to be the best, but we really want to excel at it to the Michael Jordan level. So much so that anything else is unacceptable. Remember when everybody wanted to be like Mike? What if your role was to be Phil Jackson? Wow! He went on to say they both have rings. Phil was an amazing coach. In fact, eleven of his thirteen NBA titles are as a coach. He has the distinction of having the most combined championships. The lesson we need to grasp here is, do not stop playing because you are not in the position you wanted most in life. What stops you from being the best Phil Jackson? If the aim is to get a championship ring, then you can coach your way to it and truly be influential while doing so. The experience you gain on your journey will give you the wisdom to guide someone through their season, and you both could excel.

I would like to layer onto that. In January of this year, my friend Jenai turned 33. He said this is his Scottie Pippen year. In case you are not aware, Pippen's number was 33 when he played for the Chicago Bulls. Jenai would assist his friends in getting to the next level all year long. At the time, I thought that was commendable. When you look at the statistics for the six hundred and ninety-one games that Pippen played with Jordan, you see his massive contribution to the Bulls and the six NBA rings come into the light. What is interesting to me is that his assists in the league dropped for the two years that he did not have the scorer extraordinaire to pass to. Can you imagine having someone volunteering to be Pippen for you? Better yet, who can you be Pippen for? I think it is incredibly important to be self-aware. When you recognize your role in the game (of life), play it to the best of your ability. Identify a need you can fill in someone else's life. Manage the relationships well, rest assured the team will win.

The research for this book was qualitative and utilized a loose mix of a case study and phenomenology. Qualitative because I was interested in telling a story about a specific phenomenon that would be generated by words and not numbers. A case study approach allowed focusing on context and dynamic interactions because the interpretative nature of qualitative inquiry allowed for revisiting of stories using an emotional intelligence framework. Parts of the data collection are phenomenological because they focused inwardly on the lived experiences of the Caribbean people around whom the stories are written. Setting this book in the Caribbean is both geographic and cultural.

Hello and greetings

First time we meeting

I hope you not leaving

Just stay a lil bit

I'll keep it formal

Please just act normal

Kerwin Du Bois

Bacchanalist

Chapter One

A man has to buy his own shoes

What I love about living in the Caribbean is that going to the beach is not a vacation. In fact, any body of water is reason for a good *lime*. Or it could be a place to help you contemplate life if you need to. In some countries, it is a river, some countries a creek, some countries a sulfur spring, some countries a waterfall. I am making the distinction of saying countries because not every Caribbean territory is an island. There are over twenty-five nations that touch the Caribbean Sea, and there is Guyana, the only English-speaking country in South America. Now that we have the geography squared away let us proceed!

Most Caribbean people know that a rite of passage as a child was being sent to the shop with a list for groceries. Boy or girl did not matter. I think once you were about six years old, you were eligible. There was no specific time of day or day of the week for that matter, it was when mommy or granny needed things. The instructions were always clear, "go straight and come back quick." Those instructions meant not to play along the way, not to stop and talk to your little friends, do not veer off the path, and often times do not take a shortcut.

The nice thing about Saturday mornings in a Caribbean household for children was the opportunity to watch some cartoons. You may have contemplated that all week. Adults would have chores to do, including washing, cleaning, and cooking. In some cases, they worked during the week, and children had a full week of school. This one Saturday morning, I had to be about seven, as soon as I sat to watch BraveStarr, and began to sing the catchy theme song, "Eyes of the hawk, speed of the bear, strength of the puma!" I heard my mother bellowing my name. I swear she was happy to have me as I became the errand boy. The culture is different now, and my children have never gone to the shop, but at six, I used to go, in fact, I would go to the market with my grandmother, so I learned how to choose good produce. That Saturday morning, she was baking and wanted yeast. She gave me a $100 bill, and I went to the supermarket, or as we say in Trinidad and Tobago, the grocery. So I picked up the items I needed, got to the cashier, and could not find the woman's $100 bill. Somewhere between leaving home and getting there, I had misplaced the money.

I searched frantically. By that I mean, I checked my pockets a few times because I know I had it when I left home. I had to put back the items. There was a bridge I had to cross to get to Aranguez Plaza, where the grocery was. I crossed the bridge and walked down the riverbank. I told myself, "That's it, I'm never going home again." I convinced myself at that moment. "This is it, life is done, better I dead." I started having some conversations with God and hoped the

7

river would wash me away because I had no idea how to go home and tell Gemma I lost her $100. I saw this homeless guy I knew, Emmy Shirler, he lived on the street. I told him what happened, he went home without me to tell my mother I had lost the money and that I was in the river. It was a dry river of sorts. There was water but low, it never broke its banks. People would go there to skip stones and fish for guppy. It was a populated area, so it was not desolate or scary. So I just stayed there pelting stones and contemplating my certain demise.

What had to be hours later, I hear my sister's voice bawling my name in the distance, incessant and unwavering. I thought it was safer than if it was my mother, so I acknowledged her. She was on the walkover, and I could hear her in the distance. So I walked closer and saw her. "Boy, what doing there? Mommy waiting on you! Come home. Emmy Shirler done tell her you lost the money already, so you better come home now." "Ohhh, God!" I thought to myself. Remember, she was in the midst of baking, so this was something I was supposed to get and take back quickly. Things had to stop when I didn't get back. The entire baking Saturday was a disaster. I was hearing her voice from down the street as I approached, I was understandably scared. Only to get home and realize that it was just flair. On that occasion, she did not do anything. She just chastised me, saying, "Boy, we were worried! So you couldn't come home and say you lost the money? What yuh was doing? Yuh does play too much!" She was right, the money had to have fallen out when I was swinging on the bridge or doing some nonsense. It just slipped out my pocket, and I did not notice. I got to the grocery, and it was not there.

For most Caribbean people born in the 1970s and before, we understand how corporal punishment was used to keep children in line, at home, at school, and most assuredly on the streets. Any adult in the community had the authority to upbraid an errant child. Sometimes a good scolding let you know the potential to get worse was always at arm's reach. My fear of going home when I lost the money had its roots in things I had seen before that weighed on me that Saturday morning. Adults often ruled with fear. That fear was not an absence of love, though.

One time I was allowed to go to the Savannah. I was there with my friends. My mother said to get home by a certain time. That was usually before streetlights came on. We were making kites, and I got caught up. At one point, I saw my friends look up and started to run away. I wondered why they were running, then I looked around and saw my mother coming with a big stick. Licks in the Savannah, in front of everybody! Everybody. My mother was the type of mother that would beat everybody, and my friends knew that, that is why they ran.

9

* * *

West Indian parents back in the day, especially Trinbagonians, believed that the route was - have children, send them to primary school, send them to secondary school, they get a good government job, live all their life, they die. I honestly believe that is what your grandparents told your parents, and your parents believed. My dad came from Tobago bare feet. He had this thing he used to say – "a man has to buy his own shoes." Loosely meaning that men must fend for themselves. My parents felt that once they got their child into primary school, that was it. They were not the type of parents to question things. I say this, knowing that my next of kin was eleven years my senior, and they had done this before. That shaped my thinking about the free public school system. While I felt the free education was good for West Indian children and perhaps one of the best things to happen, there needed to be checks and balances with parents. A lot of parents left their children and treated it almost like babysitting, somewhere to send them for a couple hours until they got home. They never followed up. When we started to lose the passionate teachers, we started to lose the children. We saw a shift in the type of child in the 1990s, and the older teachers were starting to retire, and the newer teachers had a completely different approach.

I feel like I was right in the middle. I feel like I just went to primary school to learn the basics – the alphabet, nouns, verbs, pronouns, multiplication tables, just whatever you need to get to secondary school. No extras. I got to secondary school. While in secondary school, it was a cool time for fashion. I felt like getting to high school made me a big man. My mother managed that thought for me for about a year. First, I was in short pants, we actually had the option to wear long pants, and I wanted that. Part of the excitement of going to secondary school was that you no longer had to wear short pants. All my peers were in long pants. My mother did not share that sentiment and would dress me for my entire first form year, and she used to ensure that I wore a marina - wife-beater, tucked into my underwear, then she would put on my shirt, my pants, belt – had bored a hole in the belt with an icepick! My mother believed in dressing me up until form one. Going into form two, my mother was still trying to dress me. I remember my mother oiling my foot and sending me out! Knees used to be shining in assembly.

While my father believed that a man had to buy his own shoes, I got shoes for school. When my peers had family living abroad and sending them high-top Adidas, and Jordan's, and Travel Fox, I did not have that! I had one Flame that I had to go to school in, that was a plastic Flame that had Scotch tape on it because my mother was not buying new sneakers until the new term. That fueled my sense of self-awareness and drove me to my first entrepreneurial venture – a fruit stall in the market. In secondary school, I had some good side business happening, and I was in with my peers. I started to experience some popularity from then. I was cutting hair and had an ice-cream parlor. My dad basically left me alone until I wrote CXC. He was well-respected in the community, by both good and bad. He helped good guys stay that way and helped to reform the wayward ones who were imprisoned. He had a career in the prison service and was a Reverend with active missionary life. He was closer to my sisters because they were older, and one of my sisters was old enough to care for me when my parents traveled.

Shortly after I turned eighteen, my mother presented me with the manifesto. The Leonard O'Reilly Callender manifesto – nobody is to live in my house for free. My father made a call and got me a job in the prison service. I was instructed to go get a haircut – I was cutting hair, but I was to go to a specific person to get a haircut, wear a white shirt, a tie, any color slacks, and head to Golden Grove to meet his best friend. I was to have all my documents in a manila envelope and a knapsack. I would start training to become a prison officer. In my dad's mind, it seemed like the next logical step. I complied...up to a point. I got the haircut, dressed, left home with my documents, and got into a *maxi*. Golden Grove was about fifteen miles from home. While in the maxi, I had a vivid and forceful reflection on the few times I had been to the institution with my dad and recounted the interactions from people being trained and how young recruits were spoken to, and in that moment, I could see the instructor shouting at me, and I would have to respond loudly "Sir! Yes, Sir!" This was about eight miles into the trip. I was more than halfway there. I pressed the bell to get out of the maxi at Curepe Junction. I don't know if it was God or the Devil, but I got out. Mind you, my dad's friend was expecting me at 8:15 that morning.

I had no idea what I was going to do. I knew what I did not want. When I walked to the plaza close to where I stopped, I saw a sign for Ann's Barbershop. I went in there to ask if she was hiring. I had been a practicing barber for a bit now. It was Monday morning, she said to bring a muse on Saturday so she could judge my ability. I had the entire week to think of how I would earn my keep in the house because I now had to buy my own shoes – literally. I went to Farida's *roti* shop nearby and sat there contemplating what to do. Hours passed. It was 1994, and I did not have a cell phone. Once I had built up enough courage, I went to my sister's house. I told her what happened. I was supposed to go see dad's friend this morning at Golden Grove...she jumped in mid-way, "What?? And you ain't go? And you by me?" She started to backpedal. She knew my father would not be pleased. She was also defiant, so she regrouped and

13

said, "Well, if you don't want that, he will have to understand. You don't want that for yourself, they can't force you." So she took the initiative to call my mother. My mother said, "All yuh have to talk to all yuh father!" My sister said, "Wait, and when daddy came home, we would call him." She did. The conversation started off cool, "Terrin is by me, he didn't..." he retorted, "he never go to...?" At this point, I'm hearing the heavy voice through the phone. The next thing I heard was, "Well, he better stay there!" That was it. My father said I was not to come back in his place, I embarrassed him.

I was in limbo for about two months. I stayed at my sister's until my mother softened him up, and then I was back in the house. He was not speaking to me, but I was back home. I had gotten the part-time job at the barbershop, so I was doing that. That was going well. About a year and a half later, my mother's house was starting to get crowded with clients because I would trim there too. I don't know if it was God or the Devil again, but a furnished barbershop had become available by default not too far from Ann's Barbershop in Curepe Junction. The previous owner could no longer afford it and was selling as is. The landlord wanted four months' rent in advance. My father paid. For me, it was a sign of support, they trusted me and helped me solidify my decision, I always knew I did not want to work for anybody. Definitely not in the government. I was never interested in being a policeman, fireman, none of those things. I always felt as though I could have made money outside of getting a government salary. I used my defiance as a catalyst to excel, you cannot be defiant and a failure at the same time. Your desire to succeed can be fueled by your defiance. I was sufficiently self-aware to understand that. I did well at barbering because I chose it and was determined to make it profitable until I decided what I wanted next.

Chapter Two

Defining Emotional Intelligence

There has been a lot of talk about intelligence, perhaps from the time, we started testing and trying to separate each other. Emotional intelligence, though, first appeared in 1990 when Peter Salovey and John Mayer wrote about it. It was described as a form of social intelligence. The rational component of human behavior (intelligence) has long been given priority over the irrational or emotional component, and consequently, the role of emotion has been less understood. Emotional intelligence is concerned with feelings and interaction. Salovey and Mayer defined it as the ability to monitor one's own and others' feelings and emotions, to discriminate among them, and to use this information to guide one's thinking and actions.

Emotions vs. Feelings

While consensus does not exist in the scientific world on a definition, emotions are a physical state that occur in response to external stimuli. Emotions are bodily reactions. Emotions, therefore, occur prior to feelings. Emotions can be observed by looking at someone. While they are often used interchangeably, emotions and feelings are not the same. Feelings are things we sense. Feelings come with thoughts. Emotions are a result of chemical reactions. They can be hidden. It is possible for a person who is depressed to hide the sadness they feel with a constant smile. The basic emotions are happiness, sadness, fear, disgust, anger, and surprise. Many of the feelings we experience can be placed into one of those umbrella categories. Learning to identify, understand, and describe those emotions is helpful for the management necessary for the interaction of the self with others.

Surface acting

In some organizations, employees are required to act in a specified manner toward customers. The actions require employees to change their outward appearances, such as facial gestures, motions, and voice intonation. This is known as surface acting. Surface acting could have negative effects on employee job satisfaction. The disconnect between their true feelings and the surface acting could lead to emotional exhaustion and burnout. One instance where surface acting is necessary and almost unavoidable is where language and cultural barriers exist. Surface acting is used to show empathy. In cases where there is a disconnect between the employee and the customer, the interaction could be frustrating for both involved. In the service industry, where employees are sometimes exposed to less than favorable interactions from customers, having organizational stressors such as policies, systems, and structure leads to emotional exhaustion.

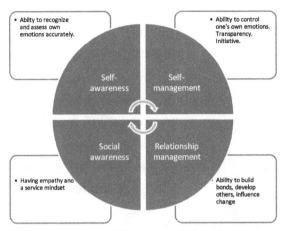

Fig. 1. *Components of Emotional Intelligence*

The first set of feelings an emotionally intelligent person recognizes is their own. They understand the emotions, they can identify them and manage them. They apply that same ability to the social circle or situation within which they find themselves. That could be work, church, school, a beach fete, a river lime and so on. Emotional intelligence has also been described as a subset of social intelligence that represents three individual-level abilities related to feelings: appraisal and expression of emotions of self and others, regulation of emotions for adaptive and reinforcing mood states, and utilization of emotions for solving problems. The emotionally intelligent individual recognizes the emotions in others as well and manages those emotions for the best possible outcome. Being emotionally intelligent is not something that you shut off once you have learned it. You read that correctly, yes you can learn it.

18

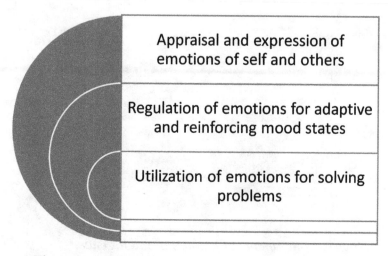

Fig.2. *Emotional Intelligence – three emotional level abilities*

It should not be confused with emotional manipulation and other negative traits that people with toxic intentions prey on, however, their ability to understand the emotions leads them to highlight those things. Emotional intelligence gives parents the ability to negotiate better with their children, almost at any age. As long as someone can be reasoned with and can identify emotions, the possibility of a rational outcome exists. Consider how many deaths could be avoided in the United States if police officers had more training in emotional intelligence instead of some of the other conditioning they are given. Consider how the culture in the Caribbean is different for police officers. There is absolutely still a line between the police and the citizenry, and there are still instances of brute force, but the fatalities are considerably lower.

The format of emotional intelligence referred to and in use, today was refined by Daniel Goleman in his 1995 work and is currently embraced by education in programs of social and emotional learning. Goleman developed a model that was reviewed in 1998 based on two hundred competency models, twenty-five social and emotional competencies that most strongly predict superior performance in many occupations were identified. These competencies were divided into five dimensions of Emotional Intelligence - self-awareness, self-regulation, self-motivation, social awareness, and social skills. Understanding the competencies is a critical step to application in daily life. After more revisions, the Goleman model of emotional intelligence appears now without self-motivation as a separate construct. That can easily be absorbed into self-awareness or even self-regulation. The competencies are now:

(1)   Self-awareness – knowing one's own emotions better

(2)   Self-management – emotional control

(3)   social-awareness – being aware of others' emotions; and

(4)   Relationship-management – the ability to motivate and inspire others by using emotions

* * *

As a dad, I recently had an opportunity to manage my twelve-year-old daughter's emotions in a serious conversation. She told me that she would like to start dating. I quickly said, "No problem, I want you to date." I was building up to get a win for myself and secure buy-in from her. I started by explaining that dating was expensive. She has a good grasp of the concept of money. She is able to assign value precisely. I know my daughter has an expensive palate and has grown accustomed to getting nice things. I explained that when dating, you have to be equally yoked in the things you do. I reminded her that she loves salmon pasta, and if she is dating, she will need to be able to afford things that she likes. Or the boy she is dating will need to be able to afford them. To afford them, she will need a job, she cannot work until she is eighteen. I might have bought myself a month before she returns to broach the subject again.

* * *

Self-control is an integral part of emotional intelligence. What does a Caribbean person with self-control look like? It is not a trick question! The answer is just like any other nationality with self-control. With all our influences, self-control may seem out of reach, however, the discipline instilled, forcibly or otherwise, in you as a child does not just vanish as you grow. That is where self-control comes from. Self-control for Caribbean people is answering Fadda Fox's "who does go to work on a Thursday or even a Friday when it have party?" with a confident – "I do." Self-control is staying committed to all your gym days, as well as laying off the roti, even the reason is to fit into your costume on Carnival Monday and Tuesday. Self-control is understanding that even if you are thinking something mean, you ought to connect the filter in your head to the one in your mouth. Self-control will not only keep you out of prison, it will help keep the peace in society. Reflect for a minute on how many things could have been different if someone had exercised some self-control. No one is asking for a constant Zen state of mind, but we may need to unlearn a few things.

Sometimes a lack of self-control can be identified in hindsight. When I was in my late teens and was on the streets constantly running the barbershop and my fruit stall, I had a pager. The distance between where I lived and where the sole office was for bill payment or customer service was prohibitive. As you could imagine, when I had an issue with service, I thought I would let them know. Typical young West Indian black boy vibes, you know the rite of passage – car with loud music, snapback, basketball shorts, Jordan sneakers, jewelry – I was on it heavy! Pulled up to the place, music playing hard outside, walked in "yeah, who is the boss in here?" I was greeted cordially, and my suggestions were heard, it actually turned into a pretty good deal because I had great suggestions to improve the service. Looking back at it, though, the approach could perhaps have been turned down a few notches, literally.

Models of Emotional Intelligence

In addition to the definition of emotional intelligence previously discussed, there are models of emotional intelligence in use that highlight different facets. There are three models of emotional intelligence – the ability model, the trait model, and mixed models that consist of both trait and ability. The ability model is the Mayer-Salovey Model. The trait model is the Petrides Model, and the mixed models are comprised of two, Goleman Model and Bar-On Model.

Mayer-Salovey Model

The Mayer-Salovey model of emotional intelligence utilizes a four-branch approach. The four branches are – recognize emotions; manage emotions; use emotions; and comprehend emotions. This model was published in 1990. In research designed to examine characteristics of perception of emotion in visual stimuli in adults, the researchers noted that in healthy people, the ability to appraise and express emotions and use them for motivational decision-making were all related skills. The researchers also found that emotional perception extended beyond facial expressions and included colors and novel graphics. The results of the research were suggestive of the fact that aspects of emotional intelligence appear to be abilities that can be measured. It, therefore, meant that the fact that qualities like empathy involve clearly defined skills, as opposed to attitudes alone, individuals with interpersonal problems may have a skills deficit that can be improved through training.

Emotional intelligence has been positioned among social and personal intelligence. Some of the principles that shaped this model included the fact that emotional intelligence is an ability and is best measured as such; emotional intelligence is a broad intelligence; it is a member of the class of broad intelligences focused on hot information processing. Hot intelligences involve reasoning with information of significance to an individual – matters that may chill our hearts or make our blood boil. People use these hot intelligences to manage what matters most to them: their senses of social acceptance, identity coherence, and emotional well-being.

The fourth branch of emotional intelligence, according to this model, is managing one's emotions. The types of reasoning included are effectively manage others emotion for a desired outcome; effectively manage one' emotions for a desired outcome; evaluate strategies to maintain, reduce or intensify an emotional response. Monitor emotional reactions to determine reasonableness; engage with emotions if they are helpful; disengage if they are not; stay open to pleasant and unpleasant feelings as needed, and to the information, they convey, complete the fourth branch.

The third branch of the model is to understand emotions. The types of reasoning contained therein are to recognize cultural differences in the evaluation of emotions; understand how a person might feel in the future; recognize likely transitions among emotions; understand complex and mixed emotions; differentiate between moods and emotions. Appraise the situations that are likely to elicit emotions, determine the antecedents of emotions, and label emotions and recognize relations among them; complete the third branch.

The second branch is facilitating thought using emotion. The types of reasoning include selecting problems based on how one's ongoing emotional state may facilitate cognition, leveraging mood swings, prioritizing thinking by directing attention based on feelings, generating emotions to relate to others, and generating emotions to help judgment and memory.

The first branch of this model of emotional intelligence is perceiving emotion. The types of reasoning expected include identifying deceptive or dishonest expressions, the ability to accurately discriminate emotional expressions; understand emotions in the context of culture; express emotions accurately when desired. Perceive emotions in others accurately through vocal, facial, or behavior cues; and identify one's own physical state, feelings, and thoughts; complete the list of types of reasoning.

The branches were from the original Mayer and Salovey research from 1990 but were modified in 2016 to enhance its usefulness. The four-branch model shows problem-solving areas of emotional intelligence. The authors noted that areas could be further sub-divided into areas of generating emotions. This revision of the four-branch model has allowed the inclusion of more problem-solving instances than before.

The Bar-On Model

Trait emotional intelligence models refer to the self-reported perception of emotional and social abilities. The Bar-On model of 2010 is the most widely used and examines a cross-section of emotional and social competencies. Bar-On described them as non-cognitive capabilities. Cognitive capabilities are involved in the act or process of knowing. They include the capabilities of perceiving, recognizing, conceiving, and reasoning. This model has been used in research on coaching intervention on the emotional and social intelligence competencies of leaders in financial services and includes five areas – Intra-personal competency, which allows for self-expression of thoughts and feelings constructively. Interpersonal skills are another included competency, which refers to how people relate to each other. Stress management, adaptability, and general mood are the remaining competencies.

The Petrides Model

The Petrides Model came to prominence in 2009 and is the second model built on trait emotional intelligence. When utilized for research among students where they examined scholastic success beyond that attributable to fluid intelligence and personality trait, the Petrides Model appeared more promising because it was more comprehensive than the Bar-On Model. Researchers studied the role of trait-based emotional intelligence of leaders in cultivating the attitude of commitment amongst subordinates in the information technology sector in India. They found that the nature and manifestation of emotional competencies differed across hierarchies. Trait-based emotional intelligence in leaders was not potent in fostering higher levels of continuance commitment or normative commitment. The nature of the job designation could be crucial to the organizational commitment affected by emotional intelligence. The mode of communication between leader and follower in the information technology sector is predominately impersonal and dominated by emails, not leaving much room for emotions.

Goleman Model

(1) Much of what is commonly known about emotional intelligence has been popularized by Goleman. Utilizing the mixed model of emotional intelligence, the components are Self-awareness, this refers to recognition of one's own emotions

(2) Self-management, the management of one's own emotions

(3) Social awareness, understanding how to interact with others; and

(4) Relationship management, managing one's emotions as well as others

An emotional competence is a learned capability based on emotional intelligence that results in outstanding performance. Goleman pointed out that emotional competencies build on each other in a hierarchical manner, one must be mastered before moving on to another.

Measuring Emotional Intelligence

Assessment instruments have been developed to measure emotional intelligence, they also have the predictive ability and ensure validity and reliability. The ability model utilizes a self-report instrument known as Wong and Law Emotional Intelligence Scale. That scale includes items that

28

refer to the perception, understanding, and regulation of one's own and others' emotions.

The Mixed Model or Trait Emotional Intelligence model differs from the Ability Model. A questionnaire is utilized to assess tendencies rather than performance tasks. There is also a self-report measure that forms a part of the assessment. The Wong and Law Emotional Intelligence Scale was developed in Asia with English as the official language. There has been interest in using it in different countries. There must be adaptations to allow for the difference in culture and to ensure validity based on the original intention of the instrument.

Leadership can be both rational and emotional. This involves both sides of the human experience – the actions and influences based on reason and logic, as well as those based on inspiration and passion. In an effort to garner a deeper understanding of how emotional intelligence affects leadership, Segon and Booth measured emotional competency using the Emotional Competency Inventory (ECI). Their intention was to test for ethical management and to ascertain whether a manager could be emotionally intelligent but morally incompetent. At the center of the framework that was utilized was ethical management, which comprised ethical knowledge, virtuous behavior, and genuineness. Within the framework of emotional intelligence competencies – self-awareness, social awareness, self-management, and relationship management, each competency now included an ethical component. After reviewing a number of cases, it was found that it was possible for individuals to display emotional intelligence competencies and behave unethically. The researchers proposed a variation of the Emotional Competency Inventory framework. Ethical Management should be a mandatory competency cluster at the heart of the framework. If there is a conceptual understanding of ethics, it would inform intra- and inter-personal practice, this would, in turn, be manifested in virtues like integrity and trustworthiness.

One of the things that studying emotional intelligence has shown is that people deal with emotions differently. In 2016 following the situational judgment test method, a large pool of forty-six workplace scenarios was tested over a number of studies to cross-validate them. The measure termed NEAT (North Dakota Emotional Abilities Test) was developed. After five studies to rationalize abilities, some limitations noted were the use of self-reporting in instances of job stress, which may be appropriate, but job performance could be reported by someone else. In light of this, there could be an opportunity for scholars to work on the development of a scale that measures emotional intelligence in Caribbean work scenarios, as well as situations outside of work because the influences are different.

Come leh we lime, lime,

Leh we lime on de corner

Leh we drink on de corner

And watch de girls passing by

Come leh we go down de road

With a drink in we hand on de Avenue.

Machel Montano

On the Avenue

Chapter Three

After work lime

What I love about living in the Caribbean is that you can drink alcohol on the streets. This is not limited to carnivals or cricket matches alone by any stretch of the imagination! Unlike the United States, where standing on a street corner drinking alcohol is not only frowned upon, it is prohibited; no such thing exists in the Caribbean. You could be having a drink upstairs at a pub on Broad Street, and a friend hails you from the street. You are most likely to head downstairs, drink in hand and talk to them. You will probably invite them up to join you at some point. If you were on Main Street, you were probably on the bridge *liming* anyhow, drink in hand and watching the world go by. After classes, or before, or whatever…many people have stopped at UG Road & Fourth St., at Big G. In fact, that place is the stuff of legend. If you know, you know. I only realized how iconic it was when a Saint Lucian, former Hugh Wooding student, asked me if I ever used to lime at Big G! I think my response was, "How you know 'bout Big G?" negated any plausible deniability I might have had. While all of this may be culturally appropriate and seen as a rite of passage in the region, it begins to get tricky and requires some massaging and perhaps proper management when you work at specific places. First, you really should not do it every Friday, or if you go to the Gros Islet Street Party every Friday, be circumspect. You should probably not be closing it down in the wee hours of the morning, still in uniform.

If you work at a reputable banking institution, and most of them are, you perhaps had to jump through a few hoops to get in. You had to have good grades, have a certain appearance, and then you get to wear the iconic uniform. As a desirable woman who works in that institution, you were probably drilled at home, and you extol the virtues of being a 'bank girl'. That perhaps makes you standoffish and out of reach for men at the institution. Your parents may be aloof, and you may not have had the close relationship with your father that others do. In a case where parents may have been focused on the image you need to uphold for the family's name, there may not have been sufficient listening to the children. They were not there to intercept when the child was going astray. That lapse in attention makes you the perfect candidate for a man who works nowhere and has all the time in the world to woo you and shower you with attention. The type of attention comes from his drive to elevate himself out of the current position in which he finds himself. He meets you at a bar on the Avenue. He is attentive and attractive because he has taken the time to understand what would catch your eye. So he is a little street, with enough polish to get a conversation going – you like it. Now, this is not the bar that your peers are at. They are on the other side of the street at the uppity bar.

You happen to find yourself on the side of the street where men are outside with beers in their car and loud music jamming. You are outside liming after work and drinking on the street to relieve yourself of the week's stress. He may have been calling out to you for a few days or weeks in succession. He may have come into the bank on the odd occasion. Now you are both on The Avenue – together. Weeks go by, then he needs to level up because he is talking to you and requires a certain look. He has always had a dream and would be much closer to it if you could help him get an SUV. He would be able to share your transportation responsibilities. He could pick you up for work some days and ease that strain. He could get you after work. He could go to the beach with you on weekends. It is beginning to sound plausible and cute at the same time. You know quite well, he works nowhere. He never had a loan from the bank. You take God out of your thoughts and co-sign on loan. Things go well for the first few payments, then the bank is looking for you and at you. You are stressing because he has another woman pregnant, and you do not understand how your world is crumbling.

Emotional intelligence has a positive association with quality of work, the capacity of work performance, care in handling company property, ability to get along with others, attendance and punctuality. What could you have done differently? How exactly did you end up at the bar on the wrong side of the Avenue, covering the bank's logo but leaving the iconic colors of the very recognizable uniform exposed? What are the flight responses we need to teach our young women? How do we get them to be discerning without being snobbish or judgmental and avoid sure pitfalls that lead to heartbreak, disappointment, embarrassment, and often a closing of the gates after the horse has bolted? It is a lot to unpack, but I am sure you see the trend and hopefully how it could have been halted before it started.

Chapter Four

Learning social awareness

I think I learned social awareness unknowingly. Well, actually, before I knew it to be a real phenomenon. Remember, social awareness is one of the elements of emotional intelligence. It means that you have an understanding of other's feelings, you are aware of other people, and you know that your actions affect others.

So in November of 2002, I found myself on a flight to Guyana with Ohene. We were both in transit at Grantley Adams airport. I from Castries, and he from Kingston. There was probably only one flight back then. As long as we were flying on the same day, it may have been inevitable. On November 6th, we had lost my best friend and his little brother. We were going to attend the third memorial service at the church where Omari had served as an acolyte for several years. At the airport, we figured we were on the same flight but not seated together. Not a big deal. We were going to the same place and would end up at the same wake that night anyhow.

Sometime after we were airborne, I was jolted out of my trance, literally staring into space by someone coming to occupy the empty seat next to me. The flight was about two hours, and we talked from one thing to the next, including the loud, lewd music I could hear through his oversized headphones. I remember being incredibly disappointed in the artist who had brought us some good conscious lyrics in the late 90s. Ohene defended him without apology. I remember thinking in high school that Ohene was quite defiant and should have been as afraid of his disciplinarian mother like most students were. So I didn't quite know he was such a prankster and could give such a good-natured ribbing. He told me on that flight that I would be the type of parent to stifle creativity because I would beat children for being noisy, I would pass on the pain that generations before mine had endured. Seemed a fair assessment. Neither of us have children, though, so one will never know!

Where I got my very succinct lesson in social awareness was prior to disembarking, I told him that later in the evening, I would tell the boys that he came to sit next to me and teased me mercilessly.

He looked at me most quizzically and said most assuredly, "It is not about the truth. It is about who gets their story out first." Wow, and at that moment, I realized that I was probably not winning this one. He assured me that as a seasoned traveler, his friends would know that he would not leave his assigned seat, and I had to be the one who moved. I have never forgotten that flight, and I think I became acutely aware of the intricacies of both storytelling and social awareness. That type of interaction may be seen as misogynistic or bullying in today's world, but Caribbean people are really not troubled by tantalizing.

Now when my sister starts a story about us having pets as children with, "Lendy, tell them how you killed the monkey," I completely understand that when I tell it, there is less shock and awe that completely underscores the fact that as a teenaged girl getting your chores checked off was job one. It really added to my social awareness and relationship management arsenal.

My formative years growing up in Guyana were filled with many experiences of having exotic pets in the house. My paternal grandfather was a birdman. He always had a towa towa, then my great aunt had a macaw named Laura. Guyana is vast – 83,000 square miles vast. My big brother is an electrician who worked in the interior at a sawmill. The distance from home was prohibitive to daily travel. As a result, the employees who lived far away did some weeks at the site and would have a week off to go home. He brought us a turtle and told us what we had to feed it and how to care for it. I remember him asking me if I wanted a monkey, and I clearly thought it was a good idea at the time. He said we would need to keep it on a chain. Small monkeys are agile and cunning. It may not have been a good idea to let it loose. I was still thinking, "Good idea."

We lived in Georgetown. The house had a clay brickyard, paling stave fence with two gates – one pedestrian and a double gate where Daddy would park. The house was concrete and wood – Guyana has a vast supply of timber. The ground floor housed the kitchen and living room. If you faced the house from the front, an enclosed staircase led to the second floor on the right. Straight ahead, at the top of the stairs, there was a double door that led to the verandah. It was a concrete verandah with wooden uprights. It was probably about ten feet long because It spanned the length of the room I shared with my sister. We had a pulley line for clothes from one end of the verandah that ran along the back of the house ending outside my parents' room. The staircase veered left a little to the second floor to the bedrooms, study, bathroom and TV room. At the end of the corridor and to the right, another enclosed staircase led to a tower. It was probably about twenty by twenty and had glass windows on all four sides. That gave us a fantastic view of the neighborhood whenever we were able to go up there.

The monkey would be kept on a long thin chain on the first set of stairs when you get into the house. It was confined to that area. One Saturday morning, in doing my chores, I had to scrub the stairs, which meant moving the monkey, free of all encumbrances. I chained it to the door of the verandah and closed the door. It was outside on the concrete. In hindsight, I do not think that I considered or perhaps even understood the intensity of the tropical heat. When I went to retrieve it, and how long the process took is foggy to me now, it had perished. I was distraught.

* * *

When I reflect on some of the things my mother did to me as a young man, I am sure I am traumatized. We lived in a cul-de-sac, and because the land was graded, the houses on the right side of the street were higher, and the stairs were outside and above street level. The houses on the opposite side were entered at street level, and you descended into them. Our house was high. The stairs were in two sets, winding around the house, with a sliding door. This was right around when the houses started becoming modernized. My mother would sit in the gallery. It was on a hill with a beautiful view. Any taxi that came, from her vantage point, she could see which of the three neighboring houses the person was going to. I was a little older, still in my teens, but after CXC, still not eighteen yet, but I was allowed to do things. At that time, my mother did not understand the new world, she used to travel a lot with my dad, and my sister was my primary caretaker. They had a great relationship, and my sister would intervene on my behalf to have her cut me some slack. She was my buffer.

My mother loved Patience, so she would sit in the gallery with a tray, have her tea or whatever, then move the tray to the side table and sit there to play her cards. From her vantage point, if a taxi pulled up, she would have a clear view. She could see where the visitor was going. A friend was coming to meet me, and I was getting ready to go out with her. She took a taxi to meet me at home. She had to have lived nearby. I know my mother would never have allowed a girl to come from far. She was tall. I remember hearing, "But who is this God Horse coming up my step here?" I just heard my mother's voice, and I am now walking towards the window to pull the curtain. I see the girl's face drawn in, walking up the steps, looking so sad and depressed. I was ashamed. I wanted the earth to open up. My mother cared nothing! Do not feel that she was about to say sorry or anything. Nothing. My mother's attitude as she turns her solitaire cards slowly and deliberately is one of stoicism. She directs the next question to me, "That person come to you?" I am thinking to myself, this woman is insane!

Now when I make jokes about the things she did to me with her, I tell her she was abusive, and she just tells me to be quiet! She always asks if she ever abused me, reminds me that she did everything for me and gave me everything. She even lets my daughter know that the things she would get away with saying to her now, I could not dare try those things. It is inconceivable for my daughter when my mom

41

says, "You feel your father could have talked to me so? All now so, your father would be nursing a wound!"

I'm a stranger

Said a pretty gal

I came down here

For the carnival

(soca) music have me in a trance

Want to play mas

Teach me how to dance

Buy a little rag and put it yuh pocket

Buy a little flag that's the way we do it

Find yuhself a band

And find a good position

When the music blast

You'll find out how to play mas

Shadow

Stranger

Chapter Five

Multi-cultural experiences

What I love about living in the Caribbean is that we have more holidays than workdays! Well, it feels that way. The beauty of living in a true multi-religious, multi-cultural country is that it is a great example of diversity and tolerance. In any of our countries, you observe a holiday that is not your religion or your culture. The inherent respect for others built into that model is commendable and teaches people self-awareness and relationship management values without shoving them down their throats or using a big stick. Organizations are also not warding off litigation because people feel slighted. You may have had the good fortune of celebrating Christmas, Diwali, Eid-al-Fitr, Spiritual Baptist Day, Whit Monday, Heroes Day, Feast of Corpus Christi, in addition to New Year's Day, Independence, and Republic Day. Caribbean people do not complain about holidays. It is just not our laissez-faire attitude to seek out additional days to work while at home.

That being said, though, the same Caribbean people use that good multi-cultural training and apply it when they move to a First World country that observes way less holidays. They learn to navigate having to get to work on time in a blizzard, with a foot of snow on the ground when they easily would not have gone back to work on the odd afternoon that they went out for lunch and it started raining incessantly, and there was no way to get back to the office.

Emotional intelligence allows you the latitude to avoid assessing every emotion that you encounter to shreds. You now possess the freedom to get out of your head because the tools you have been given allow for allocating information into proper places. It can reduce your stress level immensely and bring freedom. This is how you show up to work or that social gathering without a chip on your shoulder. Emotional Intelligence is an important skill and useful tool that can be very beneficial to the growth of both the individual and organization when understood and properly utilized. Sometimes people make a decision based on how they feel as opposed to what was logical. There is nothing wrong with passion or emotion, but it should be understood.

Years ago, as a young professional, I worked in a factory in Saint Lucia. I think that really perpetuated my love for service to others and my understanding of the concept of resilience. Many of the women who worked in this factory were school dropouts and made ends meet with the little that they were making. They also lived life fully. Their social lives always seemed way more exciting than mine. They worked five days a week and fully utilized the weekends. It was certainly an exuberant time.

A government agency was tasked with seeking investments that would benefit the island. Investment Promotion Officers would attend conventions overseas, invite investors to visit the island, cold call potential investors, all to attract a company willing to move their business in exchange for what the island could offer. The factory was invited to Saint Lucia in the 1990s at a time when the government was looking for alternatives to the fledgling banana industry. They began inviting companies to Saint Lucia with the promise of lower wages and tax incentives. This makes it attractive to international companies to establish business overseas. They pay lower wages and fewer taxes. The country was a safe space politically and a tourist's paradise. They, in turn, would provide employment for locals and, by extension, help build the community in which they operated. In the early 1990s, the factory opened in Saint Lucia and became the labor arm of an American company that expanded into Saint Lucia in a mutually beneficial arrangement. Saint Lucia provided the company with lower labor costs, lower taxes, the ease of an English-speaking destination and a factory shed housed in the Free Zone. The Saint Lucia Free Zone is an area that allows for the importation and storage of goods into the island that is specifically for transshipment purposes. No customs duties are charged on the items.

Employees are able to make a living with a consistent paycheck. The government is able to generate revenue, the employer pays income tax for the employees, and while they may have negotiated for a tax-free incentive for the business for the first five years of operation when they started paying taxes, it was significantly less than operating in the United States. That is a win for both parties. It fits the parent company's goal of making a profit. The reduced cost of labor is a significant saving.

Being a factory worker calls on a depth of knowledge and cultural practice that others take for granted. One primary one is having the discipline to do repetitive tasks. Another is time management.

There was a training process during which employees were taught to read simple schematics and assemble electronics. After some time, usually within three weeks, increased dexterity was expected, and the number of items produced in a day was to be above the established minimum. There were no immediate consequences for low production. However, if there were a turn in the United States economy that required a reduction in the labor force, the lowest performers would be terminated. In the Caribbean, the United States is seen as a dream country to live in. The images that are fed via television show sitcoms with big cities and bright lights. People attend parties, have regular dinners with their family, and life looks like a dream. The pride of saying that you work for an American company and that your work is shipped overseas is indelible.

When I started working there, I looked for ways to improve efficiency and motivate people to do more. One of the things we instituted was incentive-based production, and truth be told, it exceeded my imagination. Failure to get up to speed quickly resulted in earning just the basic daily wage and no bonus for surplus production. Setting targets early during the training period served as a motivational tool. From that experience, I believed that people could be motivated by money. However, I think there are other related factors. In the case of the factory, being competitive among peers and being able to let their hair down on Friday after going to the bank was impetus enough.

I used that opportunity to encourage those who wanted to further their education to do remedial training and provided extra lessons in my area of expertise. I spent several hours a week after work teaching some of them to read. I also solicited the assistance of my colleagues. That exercise helped build morale and narrowed the gap that existed between staff and management. I am able to see a correlation between emotional intelligence and increased productivity. Having frequent conversations with staff about their family, community, and personal interests helped them feel seen and allowed them to reach out when they felt the need.

Employees at the factory are happy to be a part of something bigger than themselves. When there is a new development in the American construction industry, devastation with floods or hurricanes or any kind of growth or destruction – including war, the product will be needed. To be a part of an industry that continually expands and innovates means that work, though repetitive, is not monotonous. The schematic diagrams change, meaning that an employee gets to do something different at every point along the assembly line. The same cannot be said for someone in another local factory that manufactures beer or underwear.

Managing Change

The link between effective change and improved performance can entail meeting organizational change through creative influences. An organization's improved performance depends on the style of the leadership.

Organizations are not limited to formal, corporate institutions. Include your family unit, the house of worship, the friend circle, and so on. Leadership styles that embrace creativity are more likely to help propel the institution towards remaining or becoming a worthy industry competition. A man needs to see himself as the king of his domain. Whatever his space is, he can wield influence. As the Jamaicans say, "Dance ah yaad before yuh dance abroad." This means, do well where you are before you attempt to make changes on a grander scale. For us, in this sense, and using the framework of emotional intelligence, starting at a tender age, perhaps in the home, can create wonders in a short space of time because the approach will be multi-layered. Transformational leadership is one of the styles that lends itself to the growth and change management style of management. A transformational leader supports an environment that fosters creative identity. This leader can use interpersonal motivational assessments to determine the appropriate human resource groups for a specific creative cluster. Institutions that use creative influences to meet an organizational change to be competitive in a dynamically global economic-based society will experience definitive restructuring or rebranding on a multiplicity of levels.

A good example is your favorite radio station. Think of how the stations in your country responded to the global pandemic that started in 2020. Did the station revise programming to adapt? Did the creative minds at the station lift the spirits of the listeners daily with new inspirational programming? Was the branding revised to be encouraging? Perhaps this would be a good time to take a deep dive to see and understand that change does not necessarily come from those with titles. Change is orchestrated based on where you stand. You can have influence without money or power. Ask a politician who just won a seat – the people have the ultimate power. We ought to keep that top of mind. Operating from a creative space gives you the latitude to craft change for yourself and others by being relentless in the pursuit of your vision. Sharing the vision with others creates buy-in and builds a groundswell necessary to move the world while standing in the same spot.

Globalization is the last stage in a constant process of official change. The speed of that change is constant and quicker today than in the past. Now, for example, it is not uncommon to see an individual change occupations in his lifetime, whereas before, the same occupation was passed down from generation to generation. Being a cobbler, for instance, was passed down for generations, as was a farmer or even a police officer. The advent of globalization following industrialization – where the means of production became mechanized and required a new set of skills and training and even cultural change, has now brought even more change.

Modernization refers to the period after industrialization. Here, third-world countries found a new way to produce and develop and adapt to the change that their more developed counterparts enjoyed.

Globalization saw the growth of the services sector. This did not exist before as there was not a need for it. Now that production was no longer as intense and strictly manual labor, there was a need to get the goods to the consumer, wherever they might be. This created the need for services like transportation, packaging, marketing, customer service, and the new, but accompanied the production and created employment. It required a new set of skills and training and put more people to work. The evolution continued, and today many plants are automated. The skill-set required for work is based on the use of technology. Entrepreneurship is high, and a lot of it is based on technology and on social media.

Globalization, by nature, spans different cultures. A manager who can adapt and flourish puts themselves in good stead. Intercultural competence is the ability to function effectively in another culture. This competence includes three dimensions - perception management, relationship management and self-management. It addresses how a manager placed in another culture in a leadership capacity sees their ability to lead others, how they value their relationship with others and how they conduct themselves. There is an element of emotional intelligence included there. Previous research on expatriates assigned to organizations found the three dimensions to be critical indicators of success and style. Within a global context, the leader becomes the face of the organization and their personal conduct becomes attached to the business and is taken as the business culture. If a leader was able to interact with the nationals in the host country and participate effectively in activities, it enhanced their self-esteem and ability to assimilate. Having a non-judgmental approach while being tolerant of differences and being willing to learn are some facets considered in perception management. Relationship management refers to relationships in general and includes interest exhibited in others, interpersonal engagement and emotional sensitivity. Self-management refers to how leaders view their personal attributes like optimism and confidence – a direct construct of emotional intelligence.

Many staff resident on islands that depend heavily on tourism as the source of income can attest to extra-regional managers. Managers who excel in these roles get involved in the culture and make the staff feel comfortable.

A global leader, among other things, was expected to interact with both internal and external clients from other countries. To this end, having a wide and comprehensive knowledge base is helpful. The use of inclusive behavior is where the leader makes decisions that impact and benefit the whole. Whole in this context is truly global as it extends from self to the organization, team, industry, and world. The leader acts nationally but thinks globally.

Several factors, including leadership and management, come into play to ensure that an organization is being run efficiently and effectively. Workplace culture plays a major role in helping to determine what leadership style is embraced and whether the direction comes from a man or woman, how it is received. The media helps shape people's perceptions of power in society, and those characteristics filter into organizations and become accepted as norms. Personality traits that managers espouse terming their success and that of the team they lead. Emotional intelligence allows a manager to bring some soft skills into their style and keep the team together while everyone perpetuates their vision.

Growth is at the center of globalization. In many industries, it is a simple argument to make that you need to expand your borders to grow your business. Globalization has caused companies to look for ways to be better than their competitors. One of the ways to be better than your competitor is by improving leadership practices. Now that the 'business as usual' adage is ineffective, leaders must adopt a principled approach to decision-making and meaningful change. Reflective leadership is gaining traction as organizations work to understand the different cultures and values of the markets in which they exist and the people that they employ and serve.

At the root of reflective leadership is change. It uses experiences and reflective learning to chart a way forward. There would be cultural shifts required at the organizational level to be competitive in a global world. The leader must be willing and able to implement them while not alienating any party that could be affected.

Organizations and workplace culture have developed over the years along with society. Magazines about work, success and growth feature women on the covers now as opposed to just men. The manifestation of that integration appears in the workplace, but it was not without a struggle similar to what existed in the wider society.

Identifying culture as a socially constructed factor that influences decision-making and relationships is an important and pivotal point in the discussion. Gender and sex are differentiated, and reference to the social ascription status is the focus. Culturally, gendered leadership across the world varies and is viewed differently by both superiors and subordinates. An understanding of both gender and culture within a leadership context can help influence social change as employees would be educated about the styles, and those expectations would be established.

Influences

The education on gender roles begins in the home and shapes how people act in society and in the workplace. As a pre-teen boy in my neighborhood, I had seen an altercation escalate that troubled me for a while. A gentleman had come by to see his son. This man was what we would call a *saga boy*. He would have his shirt open with jewelry on, he had a car with music, and he was a girls' man. He was unaware that the boy's mother was there that day. She did not live there. She saw him. He arrived with a woman in the car but came to see his son. He, too, was a young boy. So that ended up in an altercation and a bacchanal. The boy's mom said he was disrespectful, and there were some raised voices. The girl in the car wanted to come out and play. She was railing up. The boy's aunt came outside after hearing the commotion. She was obviously on her sister's side, or as Guyanese would say, she tek up fire rage fuh she sister. "Who you talkin' to? Not my sister!!" The aunt went to the back for a brushing cutlass and chopped up everybody. Everybody, like a general. That was the first violence I had ever seen in my life. I knew that was not what my family was about, so we were in awe. My mother was bawling, trying to get me back inside while at the same time trying to deter the aunt, with screams of "NOOOO!" Brushing cutlass used to be a swinging action, and she used to work for the government cleaning the roads. So she had a vast knowledge

56

of how to use a brushing cutlass. Trust me, that was a scene. It was so bad that the ambulance had to come. Everything happened right in front of the house. To me, it lasted the entire night. Looking back at it now, I am sure it could have been about three hours for the most. That is – cussing, chopping, ambulance, in that order. Those were the women I was around. They traumatized me.

As I got older, I realized that if a woman carried a trait from any of them, like how she pronounced a word or said something, any ounce of romantic interest I might have had, would be out of the door once you said certain things. A trigger is "Who you talking to so?" Every time I heard that when I was younger, it ended in an explosion. She also had a very scandalous laugh, raucous, very raucous. She was not a smoker or drinker, but she was heavy in the kitchen. She always had a food business. She would sell at construction sites. She had contracts to do that for years. At home, I would hear her say things like, "Oh, you not eating from me because you eating by your hoes and dem." She had a flair, a sort of attitude that I wanted to avoid at all costs. She would tell you to leave her house in a split second. I grew up seeing her put men out of the house. She was always around. While she was not shunned, it could be seen as toxic in today's society, but I can tell that her actions were from a place of love. She fought for her family. They are still close-knit.

The feelings that come from this type of experience are perpetuated into the workplace and on to society in a myriad of ways. The most common in the Caribbean is to shun or count out ghetto people. We often describe and associate the ghetto with impoverished living and poor levels of education. However, when a person from the ghetto achieves a level of success, it is always interesting how people want to make them a model and illuminate their drive and resilience. A lot of the ascent they face is mental, and they often do it with a quiet fire.

Wrong Address

Much has been sung about the resilience of the ghetto people and their ability to overcome. Many reggae songs are built on the resistance they constantly face. In her song Wrong Address, Etana sings about a woman who had graduated from school but had come from the wrong side of the tracks. She kept on being told, "We don't want no trouble, we don't want no trouble, no day. Lady where you come from, people die there every day." When the applicant changed her address to a more desirable parish in the video, she was looked at differently and hired immediately. That prejudice still abounds, and in many cases, two sets of people perpetuate it. The use of emotional intelligence along with education and opportunity could create different realities.

In her 1999 calypso Voices from the Ghetto, Singing Sandra with her authoritative lilt over a very melodious and punchy track tells of the plight of the people in the ghetto and the fate they seemed resigned to. The youth seem stuck there and hopeless. "Children through life keep on drifting/is either something they smoking or sniffing/maybe they trying to forget this life of misery and regret/no one to come to their rescue, except Capleton and Buju/so their boombox is their lego to drown out voices from the ghetto." In her song, the youth had normalized seeing violence, hearing gunshots, having a party one night and awake the next. They had labored and were weary. Referring to the boombox as lego is poignant. Lego is an American building block system that many children, and adults incidentally, play with and make realistic art. Phonetically, lego sounds exactly the same as a Caribbean person saying let go. The pun in that song speaks about the escape that music from the boombox would bring. Music is a sure form of expression for many depressed communities across the region and has produced many steelpan legends, instrumentalists, and vocalists. Singing Sandra was a great example of the possibilities of blooming where you are planted as she, too, had come from the ghetto and rose to the top of her craft.

How can employers unlearn the things they think they know about downtrodden people? What if they decided to employ people with the wrong address and allow them to change their circumstances and the lives of those around them by being able to be a beacon in the workplace. What can the corporate world do today, outside of beautifying a roundabout, to help elevate a community? Offering real opportunities for mentorship to those who are worthy is a small and achievable step.

An androgynous form of leadership appears to yield the best results in most cultures. Organizational structure can color leadership evaluations. Organizations are classified as either centralized or decentralized, promoting authoritarian or participatory styles of management. The organization's structure is different from the individual leader's style of management. We are aware that how your father runs the house may be very different from how your mother would run it. To this end, gender is a functional structure on which organizations are built. Gender inequality exists because of the everyday rules that the workplace abides by. Research conducted using two hundred leaders of differing ages, genders, and ethnicities used a vignette experiment where a story created for the purpose of evaluation utilized manipulated factors to elicit competent responses. The study found that because centralized companies created a mismatched context for female leaders, it was felt that female leaders should be penalized if their companies succeeded or failed. If centralized organizations performed well, female leaders were more likely to receive a negative evaluation.

On the other hand, male and female leaders were considered equally legitimate as leaders in a decentralized organization. In companies that failed, regardless of structure, female leaders were devalued more than males. The results showed that leadership in a centralized organization is a gender-incongruent role. Just holding a leadership role, irrespective of their personal style, women CEOs incurred a dominance backlash. This shows that the road to equality is still to be traveled in the workplace.

In the Caribbean, however, women have taken up the mantle of leadership and moved with a natural prowess that sees them sit in the highest offices and command the respect of their male counterparts. Women are encouraged in every sector of society. More of that can only continue to empower successive generations. Developing a leader helps both the leader and the organization of which they are a part. Specific traits are helpful to leaders, and several of them can be taught. After all is said and done, in most organizations, leaders deal with people's management and not robots. Having the emotional intelligence to deal with employees makes a difference when assessed in terms of goal attainment.

Understanding what motivates a leader can be linked to what we learn about emotional intelligence. Early psychologists would center their questions on who would lead based on ability. There is a difference between the inherent desire to be a leader versus external motivation attributed to leadership through incentives. Are people obsessed with being leaders, or do they genuinely feel it from an intrinsic motivation? Understanding someone's view of the management at the time of recruitment is important to their success and, by extension – the organization for which they work. Having a whimsical concept of what leadership entails but being driven by the need for power is not likely to make for a successful story in the end.

Businesses are impacted by several factors, including employee turnover, customer satisfaction, and product/service quality. These are, in turn, directly influenced by leadership styles. A socially conscious leader can employ any leadership style they see fit. However, it will impact the organization. Maybe we should consider how social dominance orientation and the propensity to change stereotypes could assist with cultural intelligence and cross-cultural training. Understanding the culture of the country within which a global organization functions or the culture of the migrant team members could help the global leader have a greater reach and potentially enjoy greater success.

This is an integral part of the triple bottom line approach. Globalization is encouraging us to move away from a singular management style and fuse different ones to be successful. With the continued growth of globalization, the future workforce will continue to be diverse, and it would be necessary for businesses to continue to adapt to employing different cultures and operating across borders for continued efficiencies and competitiveness. As a result, emotional intelligence is a factor that can be useful in human resource development as organizations deal with the changing workforce. Training professionals and practitioners can develop manager and employee emotional intelligence to leverage and utilize the benefits effectively.

Leadership is still a widely studied topic. Success in one organization may not hold true for another if the culture or structure is different. Many concepts can be universally applicable, but several are still situationally specific. Globalization is forcing us to think globally and act locally as our teams are becoming more diverse. Employing leadership practices that are both flexible and practical while still remaining humane, and in some cases, androgynous seems to be a good way for organizations to progress. Let us contemplate how adding emotional intelligence to that mix improves our position.

Chapter Six

Travel within the region, though encouraged and promoted, is not as seamless as the inviting posters look on the billboards in Times Square. Some islands are stricter than others. In some cases, you get your passport checked at least three times between the departure gate and the airplane stairs. That speaks of something other than a lack of trust to me, but we press on.

Knowing that there are three hundred and forty-two routes for human trafficking throughout the Caribbean in 2021 may explain why some countries go to seemingly extreme questioning procedures to protect their borders. Emotional Intelligence is an important skill and valuable tool when understood. If it is properly utilized, it can be very beneficial to the growth of both the individual and organization. Sometimes people make a decision based on how they feel as opposed to what is logical. There is nothing wrong with passion or emotion, but it should be understood.

When I was a young DJ, we traveled as a unit. At the time, we were young and in the prime of our careers. The club circuit in the islands was a booming scene, and we would be booked to do parties regularly and toured heavily. One of the guys had a love interest who would join us on this trip. She was senior to us not only by age but by experience. While she was not that older in terms of years, it showed with the way she drank, dressed, and carried herself. In those days, Alize was a trendy drink, while those of us basic dudes were still drinking rum and coke. When I first realized she was special, we had gone to a club, and she asked for a Frangelico. I had no idea what that was. I thought fancy shmancy – a Frangelico!

On this occasion, we were going to a neighboring island. We had been booked in advance and submitted our names for travel. None of us knew that she was going until we arrived at the airport for departure. It really was not an issue. We had enough room at the destination hotel, and we could double up to give him a single room. I thought nothing of it as it unfolded, but in hindsight, I understand now why the story unfolded like it did. We were all on one itinerary and passed through Customs & Immigration without a hitch. She was not booked with us and was processed separately. When we were on the outside waiting for her, our contact on the ground arrived. We waited. Forty-five minutes. An hour. Two hours.

We had the contact go ask a question. He was a son of the soil and would probably be given information. As he was returning to us, along with our DJ, so was the young lady. Our contact informed us that there had been an influx of young women coming to work in the underground sex trade, and they were being particularly cautious. She fit the profile.

They detained her for questioning. She had to explain she was traveling with her boyfriend but had paid her own way, and so on. They questioned her thoroughly but never called him or any of us to verify her identity. All these years later, I think she looked strip-ish indeed.

One way to ensure that emotional intelligence and the necessary soft skills spread throughout society would be to introduce elements of it in annual reviews. That process could start awareness and filter into training that takes place throughout the year. The vast majority of people can allow their training to transcend and transfer into their personal lives. I could, however, imagine street corner conversations discussing questions that might have come up in an evaluation! The open and honest discussions that we lack in everyday friendships would improve considerably. Men may have more genuine and heartfelt conversations with women without being labeled as toxic. Too much? Pull back? Can you imagine how the airport detention might have been avoided in its entirety if her boyfriend was able to convey, without sounding controlling, that she ought to have been more casually attired?

In many instances, growth demands change. There may be more instances of resistance to change than easy adoption. Tying emotional intelligence with resistance to change is helpful in the management of employees' efficiency during a major organizational change. To tell how both leaders and employees are doing at work, it may be a good idea to have testing regularly to look for potential gaps that could be filled by training or that may have otherwise gone unnoticed. Regular could mean a specific interval, as opposed to a high number of times. There is a model that tests twelve competencies under four domains. The four domains are self-awareness, self-management, social awareness, and relationship management. The competencies divided among them are emotional self-awareness, emotional self-control, adaptability, achievement orientation, positive outlook, empathy, organizational awareness, influence, coach and mentor, conflict management, teamwork, and inspirational leadership. Utilizing the model in 360-degree testing would provide the opportunity for self-evaluation and evaluation by others. This can be beneficial to many organizations for the growth of the employees and the business alike, and society by extension. External feedback is critical as someone may not know that they are not self-aware. While these 360-degree assessments that incorporate systematic, anonymous observations of behavior by other staff members have been found to not correlate well with IQ or personality, they are the best predictors of a leader's effectiveness, actual business performance, engagement, and job satisfaction.

♪♫

…this is my duty

To defend this artform

And be part of this beauty…

I don't need no foreign entity

to validate my identity

I could talk this thing with intensity

Me know the depths and me know the density

Lawd, we have to build it

Any gaps in it we must fill it

Anything wha' block it

We'll drill it

We have to nurture this and don't kill it

Bunji Garlin

Gift of Soca

Chapter Seven

Culture

I love living in the Caribbean because our culture precedes us and defines who we are. It unites us against the world, but we are keen to define our idiosyncrasies when necessary. If you are on Caribbean Twitter, you are well aware of how we fight each other in defense of our own little turf, but when an outsider gets on one of us, they feel the wrath of us all, like any good family. Remember when #RihannaIsJamaican was trending on Twitter? Search for it now. I promise you will not regret it. Those tweets are examples of self-awareness and relationship management.

Much of our culture is passed on by teaching subsequent generations what we learned. Our call and response type of music that came out of slavery remains one of the ways we pass on what we know. If you know anything about Grenada and their mas, they are fervent about jab jab. This form of masquerade is done in protest, as opposed to the celebratory Crop Over in Barbados or Mashramani in Guyana. In Grenada, where their branding a few years ago described them as 'land of 100,000 Jab Jabs', that to me meant everyone was involved. If you have not witnessed the spectacle of a J'ouvert morning in Grenada, put it on your bucket list. Grenadian jab jab music is distinct with the conch shell, and the drums and the lyrics often tell a story that perpetuates the culture. Years ago Synnah sang that the reason jab jab would never die is because "every nine months they multiply."

That is evident on the road when you see little children, perhaps about four years old, playing jab. The imagery of the multitudes covered in 'ole oil' – yes discarded, black engine oil; chains, animal heads, horns, and often a red-painted tongue – speaks to the commitment necessary to show up and participate in this ritual that highlights what the oppressors did to enslaved Africans. It is now liberating to show and share.

As a fifteen-year-old boy living in Trinidad, I had to ask to go to J'ouvert. The festivities start before sunrise. There could be a four o'clock meet-up to get started. My parents were of the cloth, and my mother was definitely not going to any J'ouvert to supervise me or ensure my immersion in the culture. Once her friends had satisfied her that I could go with them, they were *feters* and masqueraders, I was allowed to go. All I needed to do was stay in their eyesight, and they were good. They would go to the wire. It was an incredible experience. I stumbled back inside about eleven o'clock Carnival Monday morning. My mother did not say a word. I bathed, washed off the paint, and went to sleep. Got up about five, ate, bathed. That evening, all the boys in the neighborhood, perhaps about seven of us, had agreed to go out to watch the Monday night festivities.

We lived close enough to each other. It was a cul-de-sac. They would walk and come through a little track behind the house. We had a sort of whistle call, they would announce their arrival by a particular sound, and I would acknowledge with a response. I heard them and was dressed and ready to go.

I was heading through the door after responding. Next, I simultaneously hear a gushing sound and feel water running down my back. Unbelievable! My mother said, "Yuh wet man, dry your skin and go in yuh bed." All my friends were already outside waiting for me to go down the road. The expectation was that you would go down the road to hear music. That is what was happening and what all the young people would do. Go out, drink one Malta whole night – feel big. That dream was dashed! "You paying any rent here? Reach here eleven o'clock in the morning, sleep until five, get up, eat, bathe, and leaving? You paying rent? Go and lie down. Dry your skin and lie down."

How? Why would she wait to say all those things at night? I had been home for hours!

Stories like that lead me to believe that in those days, there had to be a manual! As a fourteen-year-old girl, I asked to go to a party held at a teacher's house. They had legendary parties, a group of boys from school had a sound system, and they were pretty popular. They were playing. Everybody was going, including people my parents knew. I say parents loosely because any night activity and granting of permission would have come from Daddy in my house. I had gotten permission and prepared to go. I think at first we were leaving at nine-thirty, which in my mind was already sounding late. I did not have a curfew. I never used to go out. My friend with whom I had arranged the ride called to tell me that her brother would take us. She was going to pick me up at eleven o'clock. I now had to relay that information to my parents.

No level of confidence, thinking downstream, and all the other things we know now could have helped in that situation. My father asked me one question, "If you leave this house at eleven o'clock, what time do you think you would be back?" I really did not have an answer. In fact, I do not think he wanted an answer. He continued, "It's Jennifer, right? Call Jennifer back, and let her know you will not be going." My father was not concerned that I had to go to school on Monday after not attending the party. He was not worried about which of his peers' children were going. I learned early in life that crying was futile. I never asked to go anywhere else at night. I think I might have attended the odd school fair or two, but that was undoubtedly in daylight.

My relationship with my father was pretty good, though, at least in my estimation. I know that I liked rap music, and one of my friends would travel to the United States every summer. She would bring back cassettes and records, and we would share them among the group of us that liked rap. Daddy would always be interested in what I was listening to. Having an English teacher as a mother, I always gravitated to the poetic style of music, so I would tell him what the songs were about as he stopped by my room whenever I was listening. I had DJ Jazzy Jeff & The Fresh Prince, Queen Latifah, Salt 'n' Peppa, Kool Moe Dee, Big Daddy Kane, LL Cool J, EPMD, Special Ed, Public Enemy, and you guessed it, N.W.A. I really liked N.W.A., they were activists in my mind, so I remember having to preface the specific track by saying, "This one has some cursing, but I think it is a really good song and the lyrics make sense to me." He didn't ban me from listening to it. I think he understood that it was entertainment and my interest in reading propelled me to it. As an adult, Daddy told me that he chose to listen to what my sister and I listened to because he did not want to lose us by not knowing our interests as a parent. He found LL Cool J to be quite the rapper. That was one of the ways he sought to manage the relationship he had with us. My sister now listens to Charlie Puth because her teenaged son likes his work, and I have watched the Trolls World Tour once or ten times because my three-year-old niece lives vicariously through Princess Poppy, and I am expected to know the references, so she does not roll her eyes or slap her forehead at me in despair.

We started by saying that culture defines us. How do we translate that into the organizations we are a part of and have it filtered back into society in a manner we can enjoy? Commerce has come a long way from simply exchanging goods and services for money. The state has ceased owning and controlling the sole means and obligations to keep social spaces in good working order. Companies are now being held accountable for their actions and are expected to practice corporate social responsibility. With this expectation, there are assumptions on both sides. Employees do not necessarily want the same things that government wants, and they are both stakeholders in the same corporation. The stakeholder assumes that the company will fulfill their expectations, whatever they may be, and the company assumes the stakeholders will be reasonable in their requests. Stakeholders are those persons or groups of people that have an interest in what happens to the company. They are different from shareholders – who have bought into the company. A stakeholder may or may not be a shareholder. Managing the expectations of the stakeholder is the task of the organization's leader. Having a socially conscious leader means having a leader who is adept enough to manage several moving parts and be accountable to many stakeholders simultaneously. Encouraging the practice of emotional intelligence can foster deeper relationships and more effective responses to potential crises within organizations.

A corporation only focuses on profit and power. A socially conscious leader has to ensure that the elements of corporate social responsibility are being met. The corporation has a legal right to pursue its interests irrespective of potential harm caused to others. This power of the corporation over society can be regulated by a socially conscious leader. In contrast, businesses that take care of their human resources, the environment and are profitable are successful. This is the triple bottom line approach to management. The news is replete with examples of shifts happening in the corporate world because of uprisings. Social activism forces companies to keep their actions above board and fair.

What are the ethical implications of consumers' choices? Business leaders can perceive and regulate emotions and could influence consumers' ethical decision-making. These abilities are components of emotional intelligence. Making decisions that also help the company assist the community and environment while satisfying the consumer makes it socially conscious. Examining the relationship between emotional intelligence and ethics in a consumer behavior setting can be considered crucial. Comprehension of the ethical decision-making of consumers has theoretical and managerial implications.

The merits of emotional intelligence and the benefits that it could provide to leaders who are expected to be socially conscious are immense. Corporate social responsibility has moved past making small donations to persons who seek them. In India, the Companies Act, 2013 mandated that banks spend 2% of their profits on corporate social responsibility projects. This can appear to be forced compliance, but it would foster support for the organization from employees who are on the frontline of the endeavor and from the consumer who also sees themselves supporting the efforts with their financial contributions.

Emotional intelligence has become a measure for recognizing influential leaders and has become an instrument for developing viable leadership skills. Given the previously discussed nature of emotional intelligence to understand behaviors in social settings and utilize the information to carefully impact others, it is easy to see how useful it could be to merge it with socially conscious leadership. There could be immeasurable gains from the deliberate act of responding to stakeholders in a way that rationalizes their behavior with the possible actions of the organization that could bridge the two.

While we will not go back as far as slavery, our culture is truly born out of how we work. The way we treat together as a community is an integral part of what shapes our emotions. Let us discuss capitalism for a bit.

Capitalism is an economic system of operation where goods and services are provided by private enterprises for a profit. There is moderate government intervention in the daily running of the businesses. Consumers expect to pay a fair price, and employees expect a fair wage for their labor. The government does not own the means of production but can provide a regulatory framework. The United States is a capitalist society - one of the best examples in the world. Adam Smith, an eighteenth-century Scottish economist, is one of the founding fathers of capitalism and released a book in 1776, "The Wealth of Nations," still studied and referenced today. According to Smith, the wealth of nations was not gold or silver but what people could get for their money. A nation's welfare hinged on what it produced. There are varying schools of thought on Smith's relevance in today's society, and some countries follow a completely different model.

Impacts of Capitalism

Capitalism as an economic system has several moving parts that work together for it to function well. At the center of capitalism is a private enterprise. These companies employ workers for their labor. Workers produce goods and services that are sold to consumers for a price. While this is happening, a government regulates the business process with taxes to subsidize healthcare and fix societal infrastructures like bridges, roads, playgrounds, etc.

There has been an emergence of new forms of capitalism known as state capitalism or refurbished state capitalism. In Brazil, Russia, India, China, and South Africa (referred to as BRICS), the state behaves like an activist and takes a pivotal role in managing economic development, employing industrial policy, financial and regulatory tools to ensure that those countries catch up industrially and technologically.

Adam Smith's Vision

Adam Smith is a Scottish-born eighteenth-century thought-leader renowned as the Father of Economics. His work has been the basis of studies by several scholars and has been built upon for over two centuries. His major work was The Wealth of Nations, a book released in 1776. In his book, Smith highlighted four things:

1. The self-regulating market
2. Specialization and the division of labor
3. Government's minimal intervention in the economy
4. The advantages of free trade

Smith believed in the laissez-faire model of economics, which would allow economies to function without intervention from the government. If everything worked the way it should, there would be equality in society with the distribution of wealth, labor, and goods. He believed that countries would be better off producing products they were efficiently equipped to and trade for those they could not produce. He was not a fan of barriers to trade. Furthermore, he was also opposed to the government giving protection to any specific industry to shield them from the competition. For Smith, an 'invisible hand' would guide the economy if everyone worked in their respective roles. He felt that social trust would guide the thoughts of the players in the market. No one wanted to see another suffer. People would treat each other fairly, and governments would have very little need to interfere. The notion of equality continued to transcend time, and we have seen revisions in how equality is approached in many areas, including food, clothing, housing, employment, and the ability to marry, among other things.

Capitalism in the United States

In the United States today, capitalism is driven by the quest for profits part of the corporation, high wages for their services from employees, and demand for a reasonable price for the products and services from the consumer. This combination, because it is largely unregulated by the government, allows for inequitable distribution across society.

Questions about whether American corporate capitalism and compassion are in contradiction still abound. Using a dated but staggering example, we see Apple's first quarter of 2012, where the $13.6 billion in sales was more than double for the same period in the previous year. The question was, "Does a company like Apple really need to make $400,000 in profits per employee and lay off U.S. workers?"

American Corporate Capitalism is a departure from Adam Smith's original approach. The American version encourages self-interest and the desire for financial success. In European economies, more social welfare programs help foster equality by protecting the poor and average citizens by redistributing wealth.

Smith believed that the efficiency of a free market would lead to a good standard of living for everyone. Competition in the marketplace would cause the production of the things that society demanded. We see that today with the constant emergence of new technological gadgets. Not so long ago, we used paper maps, then came the standalone GPS that was plugged into the vehicle, then the in-dash GPS, and now every smartphone has a maps application, and there are free ones that can be downloaded. That is one example of free-market service, and competition from others and demands from society helped it evolve. While this is not advocacy for any specific form of governance over another, using emotional intelligence from a big picture perspective could make populations more informed and help them understand their role in the process. Earlier, we alluded to the concept of the people having power.

Technology is now a significant part of today's world. Employees in our society cannot comprehend without awe how long the transaction would have taken a century ago if one tried to purchase an item like a book from another country. E-commerce started in the early 1990s. Some of the people in our workforce know nothing besides immediate satisfaction of wants and needs. Management of technology is one way to lessen the imbalance that capitalism causes. The cost of labor is one of the reasons that firms move production from the United States overseas and to China in particular. The size of China's population and their grasp of technology produce economies of scale when firms look to cut labor costs and maximize profits. However, their wage does not allow them to afford the item they produce, primarily if it is sold in the United States for a premium. Companies that utilize foreign-based labor could be made to pass on the savings to the consumer. They can build customer loyalty and market share by offering a competitive product built on features and benefits instead of features and benefits plus the price. Today's society places value on the sticker price and rates products as such. Lowering prices to make premium items more affordable would allow for broader consumption of premium goods and thereby foster equality of distribution of goods, services and wealth in the United States and worldwide.

Nobel Laureate Saint Lucian economist Sir Arthur Lewis encouraged intervention for private sector industrialization and to make small farmers more productive. Having lived in Saint Lucia for twenty years, the 'Lewis model' or the 'Dual Sector Model' developed by Sir Arthur Lewis in 1954 is familiar. What Lewis proposed was a co-existence of two sectors for the advancement of the economy in underdeveloped countries. The capitalist sector would develop by using labor from the subsistence sector, which would now be developed. The subsistence sector is managed by social norms that allow for the payment of a fair wage as the intention is not to maximize profits.

The underdeveloped world, commonly referred to as the Third World, has moved away from agriculture as the mainstay of most economies. Climate change, the cost of production, and the evolving society are some things that caused the shift. In the Caribbean, it was found that uneducated farmers who worked hard would prefer to see their children grow up educated and have prestigious careers. Saint Lucia is now dependent on tourism. Examining farmed landscapes in Saint Lucia showed that agricultural abandonment has not been limited to just former banana lands. Other crops, including coconut and cocoa, have been subject to increasing price pressures, and, more generally, the agricultural sector in Saint Lucia is struggling with an aging farmer population and growing farm labor scarcity. Saint Lucia's agricultural decline has created much economic hardship, particularly within the farming sector.

The removal of preferential access into European markets for Windward Islands bananas by the WTO has aided the decline of agriculture as the mainstay of many Caribbean economies. A liberalized trade in bananas has rendered much of the Caribbean non-competitive because the means of production was not as advanced and much of the production was natural as opposed to mechanical and chemical.

Capitalism is a good economic system. More than two hundred years have passed since Adam Smith released his book The Wealth of Nations. However, the central tenet of his work can still be applied today. Several industries that were the main focus of the work and at the center of the division of labor are obsolete today or at the very least mechanized. Technology has played a significant role in the development of many nations, including the United States. If technology is regulated a little more and standardized to narrow the gaps, especially regarding pricing and the cost of production, society could see itself getting closer to what Adam Smith originally envisioned. There are more independent nations now than in 1776, which means there is a need for trade policy, but it could be guided by the market instead of the opposite. Some nations are disadvantaged by nature because they cannot produce as much to export, but they can trade in services if given a fair chance. That way, they can also sustain their society and have a fair standard of living. The increased interest and pursuit of artificial intelligence will undoubtedly see us regress a bit to the age of industrialization, except without the people. We must learn to think about what focused machine learning, and constant automation would look like with fixed programming when produced. Have you found yourself talking to your GPS? How does that one-way discussion make you feel? If we do not stop to consider those things,

84

we will need to figure out that functionality because artificial intelligence is rising. Together, we can determine if there is room for machines to identify basic emotions and incorporate them if the programmers understand what they are.

Chapter Eight

Leaders, managers, supervisors, bosses

What I love about living in the Caribbean is that the size of our population puts us right next to decision-makers daily. I bet you know someone who everyone calls 'boss'. You know, calling someone a boss does not necessarily mean they are in charge, but their attitude may fit the accolade.

Not everyone is a business owner or has plans to own a business. The majority of people worldwide are employees of corporations, companies, or organizations in the public and private sectors. To this end, most people in the workforce are managed and led by the few who are managers, bosses, supervisors, or leaders. Is there a fundamental difference among leaders, managers, supervisors, and bosses? Or are they all created equal? Management and leadership are different, yet each is complementary to the other. Managers, by nature of their roles, tend to have a narrow focus on daily organizational tasks. They cope with complexity, set staffing structures and make long-term plans, and derive budgeting information.

On the other hand, leaders are vision-oriented, perceive the way forward for the company, and work towards achieving it. They cope with changes that could alter the vision, motivate and prepare their followers for obstacles and changes ahead and chart the organization's direction. A visionary leader can be described as one who is able to see something different when everyone looks in the same direction or at a specific thing.

Saint Lucia is renowned for the Gros Islet Friday Night street party. Remember I told you about drinking alcohol in the streets? Well, yes, every Friday! There is often a stage where with live performances from artistes, limbo dancers, and carnival bands. It really is a sort of mini-festival. Of course, there is always barbeque chicken. It used to be quite simple – barbeque chicken and green fig salad – now it is a culinary dream. Tourists and locals alike are guaranteed to get chicken prepared in a variety of ways, fish in a few combinations, as well as other seafood delicacies.

The police would set up signs to direct traffic on the narrow streets that accommodate parking and pedestrians who make their way to the vendor's area, small bars, and restaurants in the otherwise sleepy beach town. This happens every Friday night except Good Friday. Oistins is a very close second. I think they are second because MADD had sung, "If you think you know 'bout party/if you feel you know 'bout fete/'til you get to Gros Islet/man you ain't see nothing yet/so where we going and feel alright? Is Gros Islet tonight?"

Visionary Leadership

As you would imagine, the chicken and meat import business is a brisk trade on the island. There were at least three major importers that had branches across the length and breadth of the island. The optics there could have looked airtight to a regular person and prevented entering the market. Vision is what allowed Valley Cold Storage to enter the fray. The constant development of the business over the years – both in brand-building and human resource development – led to the very competitive entity that exists today with more outlets than some of the pre-existing competitors. Vision can help steer an organization in the right direction and can give them a competitive advantage.

When a business is opened in a crowded space, it must seek to understand its positioning in the area. Caring about the product is imperative. As an artiste, I believe that success and money are the by-products of caring about your craft. The same holds true for businesses and their understanding of emotional intelligence. A leader who crafts a vision will often have a roadmap for its execution. Having a thorough understanding of the people who will work there, the environment within which both the people and the business operate, relationship management, and relationship building will go a long way to ensure the brand not only survives but thrives. Think about it, this framework is relevant to many types of businesses.

As Saint Lucia continues to expand the tourism offering for both tourists and locals alike, the number of street parties in Gros Islet's have increased, as have the number of party days in the week. If you miss Gros Islet, there is always Anse La Raye, Dennery, Vieux Fort, or Laborie, to name a few. That is another thing I love about living in the Caribbean. I know you are getting the impression that there is wall to wall partying, and people do like to remind you that "I live where you vacation!"

However, in all its splendor, the Caribbean has made significant contributions to education, culture, sports, and business, to highlight a few areas. Some of our proudest moments include having three Nobel Laureates – Saint Lucia's two – Sir William Arthur Lewis and Sir Derek Walcott; and Trinidad and Tobago's Sir V.S. Naipaul. Our colonial past, still very present in the gentlemen's titles! Naturally, our athletic prowess and the world domination at the Olympics make us think the world knows the sound of Eternal Father, Bless Our Land!

While vision helps define organization's culture, it guides nations. We each believe that our country, as small as it may be in the grand scheme of things, is the best. We market ourselves separately and show up competitively.

Sometimes, we operate in a world of Rambo Diplomacy among ourselves. Black I sang about "Big fish eat, small fish," and I relate that to our pre-lenten carnivals where only the big survive and thrive. Using producers from several smaller islands allows the sound to be different and accords a universality of tone when the music hits the streets. The more we can connect and work together, the better off we will all be. For instance, if the vision of a local tourism organization is to attract the most sales from a finite market, and to gain competitive advantage, then a leader will set the direction of the organization's efforts and align people involved in the efforts to work collectively towards this vision. A leader thinks of the bigger picture while the manager works on the daily execution of the internal affairs that keep the machinery going. Yes, managers and leaders differ, but they complement each other.

A leader's job becomes easier, and they are deemed successful when creating more leaders, not by how well people follow them or how many people they lead. They can lighten their own load and spread the vision further. That requires a level of self-awareness and relationship management that fosters coaching that is uplifting.

Are you offering masterclasses in your space? Are you coaching your followers intending to create more leaders? Is your leader holding firm to the reigns of command? Are you being micro-managed, or is there a level of autonomy? These are good indicators of where change may be necessary or a growth mindset in the organization. As a leader, you are in a position to break the cycle of bad bosses. You can be different from the superior that you once had.

Leaders tend to treat their followers the same way they were treated. This proves that leadership is complex, and followers need to feel valued at whatever level in the organization. An emotionally intelligent leader can monitor their moods through self-awareness, use self-management to change them for the better, understand their impact through empathy, then act in ways to boost the spirit of those around them through relationship management.

Chapter Nine

What lenses are you using?

An interesting fact about finding a framework is that you can use those same lenses to look at other scenarios. Now that we have examined our upbringing, our relationships with our parents, co-workers, neighbors, friends, and the like. Let us not stop there. How can we apply the lessons contained in emotional intelligence to our daily lives in our own way? The concept is simple and can be taught to anyone. The onus is now on each of us to empower all of us.

As Caribbean people, we know that the good education of our forefathers without an injection of our culture makes our comprehension and application of it a little more strained. Access to the internet has made the world incredibly smaller, which is both good and bad. In some instances, it drives us to do better. In others, it makes us want without striving.

What concepts can we build on in the Caribbean and do so with an emotionally intelligent framework? As Jamaicans in the diaspora work to exonerate the Garvey name, what do you think Garveyism would look like today if perpetuated by everyone? How can Caribbean people empower themselves if they work together?

What would it look like if we considered owning the means of producing something, let us say, in a cooperative spirit? It should function with a level of professionalism like some of the best cooperatives in First World countries. Ponder on the operations of companies like Ocean Spray, Land O'Lakes, Mondragon, and REI. All of these businesses are worker cooperatives. Yes, the employees own the business. Therefore they make decisions about their operations and decide how they should look in the future. The employees share in the profits and are inextricably linked to the business being a success.

Many of the countries in the Caribbean archipelago are heavily dependent on tourism. It would be impressive to see a cooperative hotel where the employees are the stakeholders and the shareholders. It could enjoy low attrition, employees could be engaged, their own business, pilferage could be low, they could be their own public relations agents and recruit like-minded people to be a part of the business. Who is the Minister responsible for cooperatives in the current government? Do you know the government's policy of cooperative development? In your quest to manage relationships more intelligently and to do your part to create a more emotionally intelligent country, collaborative efforts should increase. Do not be shy about wanting to have discussions to pool resources. Creating a legacy does not have to be a solo event. Team sports are fun for players and spectators. Are you Michael Jordan, Phil Jackson, or Scottie Pippen? Get active. Pick a side. You may have lost enough time procrastinating. You will only lose more if you do nothing.

Chapter Ten

Self-help!

I love living in the Caribbean because we have a statement or parable for every situation! In this case, Guyanese would say, "One one dutty build dam,' or in Jamaica, they say, "One one cocoa full basket." There are small steps you can take daily to increase your level of emotional intelligence. From the stories we have told here, you can highlight the growth and the areas of awareness experienced even before knowing that it had a name.

There are few things scarier than the future. The unknown has always been made to seem daunting. However, the extent to which it could be scary may be directly related to how prepared one is to face it. The future of decision-making could become more automated. In fact, there may be decisions that should be automated for the more efficient running of society. People may view automated decision-making as removing power, but it could also be one less thing to think about. The inverse could also be true. Automating the thought process could be quite empowering. Having the tools to face the uncertainty that the future will bring will make dealing with it simpler.

This list of ten emotions you are likely to encounter in your everyday life defines them for you and could help you think about how you process your reactions when you acknowledge the emotion. One thing about emotions, they are impermanent. Treat them as such, acknowledge them when they are there but know they can change.

Happiness – a pleasant emotion, often characterized by laughter and a feeling of contentment. Happiness is not the absence of struggle, but it is believed that one could choose to be happy.

Sadness – an emotional response to something unpleasant. It could have been sudden, often associated with pain. Sadness could linger and devolve into depression and could need treatment; otherwise, it too shall pass with proper acknowledgement and understanding.

Fear – this emotional state is often driven by feelings of uncertainty and perhaps a loss of control at the moment. You could be unsure of what happens. Next, this could elicit a fight or flight response.

Surprise – this is often a fleeting emotion. It could be triggered by something unexpected and could be either pleasant or unpleasant.

Disgust – This emotion shows personal preferences. You may be adversely affected by someone else's decision to hold yourself to a higher moral or ethical standard.

Anger – This is an emotional response that could be related to a line that has been crossed. It may be personal or collective. This emotion is one that we could all learn to handle well as we grow. It could help avoid permanent damage inflicted in our temporary state.

Disappointment – could be felt if an event did not go the way you expected. This could be fleeting, depending on the situation. You could be disappointed in having to drive an additional two miles because the gas station on the corner was refueling when you were starting your journey. A longer-lasting sense of disappointment could be learning that your automaker has ceased to produce manual vehicles.

Resentment – this is a strong unpleasant emotion, often characterized by personal preferences. It is complex and often characterized by holding on to things of the past. You may harbor feelings of resentment for a demotion.

Shame – an unpleasant emotion shaped by the outside influences of society. This emotion is directly related to self-awareness and your control of that awareness. A three-year-old child may not be ashamed if their food falls on the ground. In fact, they expect to be given more. As an adult, in the Western culture, you may be ashamed if you go to a fine dining establishment and cannot eat with a knife and fork.

Trust – this is a pleasant emotion, and it is related to feelings of safety and respect. There are varying degrees of trust that can be reposed in a person or a thing. You can trust your vehicle to get you safely from place to place. It is almost second nature. In an interpersonal context, you trust your team members to respect the company's property because your standard of living is directly related to it.

Here are some questions that can be helpful on your journey to a more emotionally intelligent version of yourself and a more emotionally intelligent society.

1. What do you do for fun?
2. How do you deal with negative feedback?
3. Change is the only constant in life. How do you handle change?
4. You are always the lead contributor to a group project. Your ideas work, the rest of the team backs you, and the group looks good. How do you ask them for more input?
5. What was the last thing you failed at? Why?
6. What would you say is your biggest challenge?
7. How do you recover from a stressful day?
8. How would you handle an irate customer in your line of work?
9. What brings you satisfaction?
10. What makes you angry?

Answering these questions will help you assess your own emotional intelligence journey. It can tell you how much you know about your own emotions and help you relate that to where you need to be. You will also see how you can affect other people's emotions and manage those relationships in a social context.

Start by listening more. Listening is not just an auditory exercise. Listening is a complete cycle, you hear what is being said, or in some cases, what is not being said, you interpret it and give the requisite feedback. Listening is directly related to emotional intelligence if we look at it using the framework we outlined. You need to be able to do those things for yourself and others. Pay attention to everything that is happening around you, be present in your listening.

Some of us are great when it comes to going down rabbit holes. Be aware that you are going off the track. Stay self-aware and remind yourself of why you are venturing there. How is it helpful? If it improves the quest that got you there, then be sure to let related parties know you have taken a turn, and you may find something helpful that helps you manage your relationship with others if necessary.

Observation is a form of awareness. If you are in a situation as an observer, you have a front-row seat to a process and can make informed decisions about things that concern you and others if necessary. Observation provides a perspective that second-hand or third-party information does not facilitate. Being an observer works best when you are present in the moment. Many people have been physically present in a situation but not mentally or emotionally aware. You possess the power to change that.

Where emotions are concerned, an equal and opposite reaction is not always immediately required. It is fine to take some time to process a situation and have a delayed response that may be appropriate as opposed to being wrong at the moment and having to remedy a situation thereafter. Think about how much more confident you would sound and the other person would feel if you say, "Give me an hour to get back to you with an answer," instead of saying yes to something you are unable to deliver. That time could raise your credibility and help you hold yourself accountable for the decision you make. Do not be afraid to make decisions. Indecision gets you no points. Uncertainty indicates that your critical thinking skills need some sharpening.

Help yourself by outlining your thought process and controlling it. Now that you are familiar with being self-aware and identifying and controlling your own emotions, then extending that to others, start thinking in systems. Use a big picture approach and identify systematically what could work and what may not. Allow your full-cycle thinking to become automated and natural without going down the rabbit hole unnecessarily. Let it be as simple as getting home to watch your favorite comedy after work. You turn on the TV at 8 o'clock and fall into hysteria. You anticipate the TV will work, the cable is connected, the electricity is on, the pole outside your house is as it should be. Many things had to be aligned for your show to be aired, and they all worked together. That is how your thoughts should be. You must understand the system.

…something says keep pressing on

A voice in my head

Keep talk to me…

It tells me the road is long

It tells me we must be strong

Roll with the pain and strife

Today is the start

of the rest of your life

Edwin Yearwood

Voice In My Head

Lingo

Lime – a gathering of two or more people. There may be music, food, and drinks. It can be compared to hanging out but with way more vibes.

Maxi – short for a maxi taxi. A privately owned mini-bus used for public transportation.

Roti – a round unleavened flatbread made with flour. It has its origin in India and is popular in Caribbean countries, where East Indian food forms part of the cuisine.

Saga boy – a well-dressed man.

Feters – people who attend parties – commonly known as fetes.

Notes

The rational component of human behavior... Cho, S., Drasgow, F., & Cao, M. (2015). An investigation of emotional intelligence measures using item response theory. *Psychological Assessment, 27*(4), 1241–1252. doi:10.1037/pas0000132

Emotional intelligence has also been described as... Clark, J. M., & Polesello, D. (2017). Emotional and cultural intelligence in diverse workplaces: Getting out of the box. *Industrial & Commercial Training*, 49(7/8), 337. doi:10.1108ICT-06-2017-0040

The Mayer-Salovey Model of emotional intelligence... Mayer, J. D., DiPaolo, M., & Salovey, P. (1990). Perceiving affective content in ambiguous visual stimuli: A component of emotional intelligence. *Journal of Personality Assessment, 54*(3/4), 772. doi:10.1080/00223891.1990.9674037

Surface acting could have negative effects... Lee, Y. H., Lee, S. H. B., & Chung, J. Y. (2019). Research on how emotional expressions of emotional labor workers and perception of customer feedbacks affect turnover intentions: Emphasis on moderating effects of emotional intelligence. *Frontiers in Psychology, 9.* doi:10.3389/fpsyg.2018.02526

Surface acting is used to show… Feyerabend, R., Herd, A. M., & Choi, N. (2018). Job satisfaction and turnover intentions among Indian call center agents: Exploring the role of emotional intelligence. *The Psychologist-Manager Journal, 21*(2), 106–129. doi:10.1037/mgr0000071

Employees are sometimes exposed to less than favorable… Kashif, M., Braganca, E., Awang, Z., & De Run, E. C. (2017). You abuse but I will stay: The combined effects of job stress, customer abuse, and emotional intelligence on employee turnover. *Journal of Management Development, 36*(7), 899–914. doi:10.1108/JMD-06-2016-0095

Cognitive capabilities are… Rastogi, M. R., Kewalramani, S., & Agrawal, M. (2015). Models of emotional intelligence: Similarities and discrepancies. *Indian Journal of Positive Psychology, 6*(2), 178–181.

Research on coaching intervention…Dippenaar, M., & Schaap, P. (2017). The impact of coaching on the emotional and social intelligence competencies of leaders. *South African Journal of Economic and Management Sciences, (1)*, e1. doi:10.4102/sajems.v20i1.1460

Research among students where…Di Fabio, A., & Palazzeschi, L. (2015). Beyond fluid intelligence and personality traits in scholastic success: Trait emotional intelligence. *Learning and Individual Differences*, 40, 121–126. doi:10.1016/j.lindif.2015.04.001

Studied the role of trait based...Bhalerao, H., & Kumar, S. (2016). Role of emotional intelligence in leaders on the commitment level of employees: A study in information technology and manufacturing sector in India. Business Perspectives & Research, 4(1), 41-53. doi:10.1177/2278533715605434

A questionnaire is utilized to assess...El Ghoudani, K., Pulido-Martos, M., & Lopez-Zafra, E. (2018). Measuring emotional intelligence in Moroccan Arabic: The Wong and Law emotional intelligence scale. Revista de Psicologia Social, 33(1), 174–194. doi:10.1080/02134748.2017.1385243

Segon and Booth... Segon, M., & Booth, C. (2015). Virtue: The missing ethics element in emotional intelligence. Journal of Business Ethics, 128(4), 789–802. doi:10.1007/s10551-013-2029-z

In 2016 following the situational judgement... Krishnakumar, S., Hopkins, K., Szmerekovsky, J. G., & Robinson, M. D. (2016). Assessing workplace emotional intelligence: Development and validation of an ability-based measure. *The Journal of Psychology, 150*(3), 371–404. doi:10.1080/00223980.2015.1057096

Being a factory worker...Morgan, G. (2006). Images of organization. Thousand Oaks, CA: Sage.

Intercultural competence is the ability to function...Bird, A., Mendenhall, M., Stevens, M. J., & Oddou, G. (2010). Defining the content domain of intercultural competence for global leaders. *Journal of Managerial Psychology*, 25(8), 810–828.

A global leader among other things ...Caligiuri, P. (2006). Developing global leaders. Human Resource Management Review, 16(2), 219–228.

The use of inclusive behavior... Gabrielsson, M., Seristo, H., & Darling, J. (2009). Developing the global management team: A new paradigm of key leadership perspectives. *Team Performance Management*, 15(7/8), 308–325

The identification of culture as a socially... Ayman, R., & Korabik, K. (2010). Leadership: Why gender and culture matter. *American Psychologist*, 65(3), 157-170

Organizational structure can color leadership evaluations... Chin, L. G., (2016). Unequal egalitarianism: Does organizational structure create different perceptions of male versus female leadership abilities? *Gender In Management: An International Journal*, (1), 19. doi:10.1108/GM-10-2014-0093

A corporation only focuses on profit... Bakan, J. (2004). *The corporation: The pathological pursuit of profit and power*. New York, NY: Free Press.

In contrast, businesses that take car...Okanga, B., & Groenewald, D. (2017). Leveraging effects of triple bottom lines business model on the building and construction small and medium-sized enterprises' market performance. *Acta Commercii*, 17(1), 1-14. doi:10.4102/ac.v17i1.457

Business leaders have the ability to perceive and regulate... Chowdhury, R. (2017). Emotional Intelligence and Consumer Ethics: The Mediating Role of Personal Moral Philosophies. *Journal of Business Ethics*, 142(3), 527-548. doi:10.1007/s10551-015-2733-y

Maybe we ought to consider... Alexandra, V. (2018). Predicting CQ Development in Context of Experiential Cross-Cultural Training: The Role of Social Dominance Orientation and the Propensity to Change Stereotypes. *Academy of Management Learning & Education, 17(1)*, 62-78. doi:10.5465/amle.2015.0096

There has been an emergence... McNally, C. A. (2013). How emerging forms of capitalism are changing the global economic order. *AsiaPacific Issues*, 107, 1–8

Questions about whether American...George, J. M. (2013). Compassion and Capitalism Implications for

Organizational Studies. *Journal of Management*. Advance online publication, doi:10.1177/0149206313490028

Farmed landscapes...Walters, B., & Hansen, L. (n.d). Farmed landscapes, trees and forest conservation in Saint Lucia (West Indies). *Environmental Conservation, 40*(3), 211-221

Globalization is the last stage...Danimir, Š., Maja, C., & Daniel, B. (2014). Globalization and management. *Ekonomski Vjesnik, Vol XXVII, Iss 2, Pp 425-436 (2014)*, (2), 425.

One of the ways to be better than your competitor...Castelli, P. A. (2016). Reflective leadership review: a framework for improving organizational performance. *Journal Of Management Development, 35*(2), 217-236

With the continued growth of globalization...Clark, J. M., & Polesello, D. (2017). Emotional and cultural intelligence in diverse workplaces: getting out of the box. *Industrial & Commercial Training, 49*(7/8), 337-349. doi:10.1108/ICT-06-2017-0040

In India the Companies Act... Lawande, N. (2016). Being Socially Responsible & It's Importance in Bank Employees. Clear International Journal Of Research In Commerce & Management, 7(3), 57-60.

Emotional intelligence has become a measure for recognizing... Downing, J. A. (2016). *Emotional Intelligence, Leadership Style, and Job Satisfaction in Contrasting Workplace Environments.* ScholarWorks

Emotional intelligence has positive association with quality... Mucchal, D. S., & Solkhe, A. (2017). An Empirical Investigation Of Relationship Between Emotional Intelligence and Job Performance in Indian Manufacturing Sector. Clear *International Journal of Research In Commerce & Management*, 8(7), 18-21.

There is a model that tests... Goleman, D., & Boyatzis, R. E. (2017). Emotional Intelligence Has 12 Elements. Which Do You Need to Work On?. *Harvard Business Review Digital Articles*, 2-5.

Tying emotional intelligence with resistance to change... Malik, S. Z., & Masood, S. (2015). Emotional Intelligence and Resistance to Change: Mediating role of Psychological Capital in Telecom Sector of Pakistan. Pakistan *Journal of Commerce & Social Sciences*, 9(2), 485-502.

Management and leadership are different...Kotter, J. P. (2001). What leaders really do. Harvard Business Review, 79(11), 85-96.